Expanded

FEELING YOUNGER WITH HOMEOPATHIC HGH

The Leading Edge for Anti-Aging

Foreword by Howard Turney
The Father of HGH

By Howard A. Davis, Ph.D.

Expanded
FEELING YOUNGER WITH HOMEOPATHIC HGH

The Leading Edge for Anti-Aging

ISBN #1-884820-58-1
Library of Congress Catalog Card Number 00-130162

Printed in the United States of America
Third Printing, Revised and Expanded, February 2000

Published by Safe Goods
283 East Canaan Rd
East Canaan, CT 06024
860 824-5301

FOREWARD

You are to be congratulated in managing to formulate a homeopathic formula, which gives the results with human Growth Hormone, which previously could only be obtained by injection.

This will be a boon to thousands of people. My wife and I have been using homeopathic HGH for some time now, and I have been supplying them to my 94-year-old aunt. We are receiving all the benefits we were previously experiencing with the injectable form of HGH.

I have been taking the HGH injections for over 8 years now, longer than any other adult we know of. I have been called the "Father of Growth Hormone" by the media, based on my having pioneered the field, and have appeared all over the world promoting the use of HGH as a necessary anti-aging medication.

Our anti-aging website has made thousands of physician recommendations to those who want to enhance the quality of their lives, and retard the debilitating signs of old age.

Howard Turney
The "Father of Growth Hormone"

ABOUT THE AUTHOR

Dr. Howard Davis has done in-depth research in the health field since 1964. He has studied all areas of health, including homeopathy, nutrition, herbs, chiropractic and holistic therapies, as well as psychology and the functions of the subconscious mind.

He has focused on knowing specifically how the body works and how chemicals and nutrients affect it. He has interwoven that knowledge with an acute understanding of the body's relationship to, and interaction with, the outer world of the environment and the inner world of the mind.

Dr. Davis has also developed new technologies for cosmetic production. In addition to numerous other homeopathic products, he has formulated the first homeopathic skin and hair care line.

Dr. Davis serves on the Board of Directors of the American Holistic Health Association. He is a member of the American Academy of Anti-Aging Medicine, American Association of Homeopathic Pharmacists, Association of Official Analytical Chemists, the American Nutraceutical Association and the Society of Cosmetic Chemists.

Expanded
FEELING YOUNGER WITH HOMEOPATHIC HGH
The Leading Edge for Anti-Aging

DEDICATION

This book is dedicated to Howard Turney the "Father of Growth Hormone". Mr. Turney has dedicated his life to promoting HGH as an anti-aging modality of the first order. He was responsible for creating the first anti-aging clinic with HGH as the primary therapy. At present Mr. Turney is advocating homeopathic HGH to the many thousands who contact him. As Ruskin said; "Genius is only a superior power of seeing". Howard Turney keeps seeing into the present and the future of anti-aging therapies.

DISCOVERED: THE SECRET TO STAYING YOUNG

For decades different products have bombarded us with the promise of making us feel and look younger. What is the secret to staying young? Dare we think that we have discovered it? Quite possibly, yes, since we now have evidence that it has been within the human body all along.

Many studies have shown a direct correlation between aging and a lack of Growth Hormone. We believe this is true, and we invite you, not only to embark on a journey, but to arrive at a destination people have been searching for since the days of Ponce de León: The Fountain of Youth.

Read on and discover why Growth Hormone may be the closest thing to the Fountain of Youth ever found.

SIGNS OF GH DEFICIENCY

When we were young our pituitary gland excreted Growth Hormone which caused us to grow to maturity causing our long bone growth to be completed between ages 20 and 25. Our brain's pituitary then loses its "motivation" and instead of establishing itself at a balanced level, human Growth Hormone (called HGH or GH) begins to decrease steadily, and signs of aging appear.

Studies show that GH continues to decline as we age. Therefore, we need to increase GH in order to control or possibly reverse the effects of aging.

Consider the following illustration of the
decline of Growth Hormone.

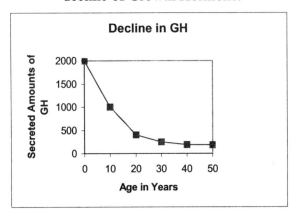

We know that, as we age, we secrete less GH. The
following can be some of the signs of its depletion:

Wrinkles, Fine Lines	Poor Memory, Cognition
Thinning Hair	Lack of Enthusiasm
Sagging Skin – Including Triceps	Slow Nail Growth, Poor Condition of Cuticles, Nails
Diminishing Eye Sight	Graying Hair
Low Energy	Skin Problems
High Cholesterol (LDL) Triglycerides	Weight Problems (Weight Loss and Weight Gain)
Slow Healing of Wounds	Poor Stamina
Cellulite	Sleep Difficulties
Immune System Problems	Disease Conditions
Blood Pressure Low/High	Emotional Instability
Failing Sexual Performance	Lack of Muscle Tone
Joint Problems	

BENEFITS OF HUMAN GROWTH HORMONE

According to research, Growth Hormone offers a wide variety of health benefits in many areas. These benefits lead to better health and a more beautiful appearance and can range from weight loss and greater muscle tone to improved sexual function.

There are many studies that show the benefits of GH. One of the most popular was conducted by Dr. Leon Cass Terry, M.D., Ph.D., Pharm.D., at the Medical College of Wisconsin, and Dr. Edmund Chein, M.D., at the Palm Springs Life Extension Institute. Using low doses and high frequency GH injections, they found the following improvements after six months to two years of therapy in 202 patients. The total average for these patients is as follows:

Strength, Exercise & Body Fat	Improvement
Muscle Strength	88%
Muscle Size	81%
Body Fat Loss	72%
Exercise Tolerance	81%

Skin and Hair	Improvement
Skin Texture	71%
Skin Elasticity	71%
Wrinkle Disappearance	61%
New Hair Growth	38%

Healing, Flexibility & Resistance	Improvement
Healing of Old Injuries	55%
Healing of Other Injuries	61%
Healing Capacity	71%
Back Flexibility	83%
Resistance to Common Illness	73%

Sexual Function	Improvement
Sexual Potency/Frequency	75%
Duration of Penile Erection	62%

Frequency of Nighttime Urination	57%
Decrease in Hot Flashes	58%
Menstrual Cycle Regulation	39%

Energy, Emotions, & Memory	Improvement
Energy Level	84%
Emotional Stability	67%
Attitude Towards Life	78%
Memory	62%

Thierry Hertoghe, M.D., at the Academy of General Medicine of Belgium, showed improvements in cosmetic appearance in another recent study of 48 people who injected a very low dose of Growth Hormone. That study showed the following results:

Cosmetic Appearance:	Improvement
Face Less Wrinkled	71.0%
Bags Under the Eyes Reduced	65.8%
Drooping Cheeks Firmer	75.5%
Double Chin Firmer	62.5%
Sagging Triceps Firmer	60.7%
Abdomen Flatter	48.0%
Aged Hands Appearing Youthful	41.6%
Bulges Above Knees Reduced	41.2%
Small Lips Fuller	25.0%
Gingival Shrinking	20.0%

Psychological Factors:	Improvement
Fatigue Reduced	86.8%
Stress Reduced	83.7%
Depression Alleviated	82.7%
Self-esteem Improved	79.2%
Mental Stability	77.8%
Anti-Social Behavior Reduced	77.8%
Anxiety Alleviated	73.5%
Confidence Improved	71.4%
Verbal Abuse Reduced	71.0%

Many people enjoy the benefits of plastic surgery to help them look and feel younger. However, we can see from the above studies that the body can improve from within—and *extend* that improvement outward—with the help of GH. GH also works great with plastic (and other) surgery because, as the research shows us, there seems to be a decrease in the amount of time a wound takes to heal.

Other studies show that GH can restore the body's ability to hydrate itself—hold water in its tissues—in a balanced form. A baby's tissues will hold about 90 percent water, which is what makes the skin soft and smooth; an adult's tissues can hold about 60 percent water; and an elderly person about 40 percent. Properly dosed GH could bring an individual's hydration back to around 60 to 70 percent, that of a 20 or 30 year-old. This is probably one reason why people using GH often report that their skin is soft and pliable and that fine lines and wrinkles fade.

HISTORY OF GROWTH HORMONE

Dr. Harvey Cushing discovered GH in 1912, and by the 1920s there was mention of GH in scientific journals. In the 1960s, endocrinologist Dr. Maurice Raben gave GH to a child who was growth deficient; the boy began growing normally. This remarkable advance was hailed around the world, but the best was yet to come. In 1962, Dr. Raben administered GH to a 35-year-old individual, and in two months the person noticed a new energy, vigor, and sense of wellness.

Also in the 1960s, in Sweden, Dr. Thomas Falkheden noted that the loss of pituitary functions produced negative changes in the body. Whether those changes were due to surgery or disease, he found that they were related to a lack of GH. At that time, GH was difficult to obtain, so studies were severely limited.

Until 1985, GH could be obtained only from human pituitary glands. Producing GH, then, was very time-consuming, and there were problems with purification. At Genentech in 1985, a team of scientists headed by Dr. David Goeddel patented recombinant, or bio-engineered, human Growth Hormone. Simply speaking, a natural plasmid purified culture (which can be non-animal) is formed and the bioengineered DNA for Growth Hormone is inserted where it "infuses" in the culture and over time develops the 191 single chain amino acids pattern that duplicates human Growth Hormone. The inert powder is removed and the rest (HGH) is freeze-dried and later solubilized for injection (or for homeopathic or oral molecular use.) This made it possible for GH to be more readily available. Other pharmaceutical companies have since developed their own versions.

In 1989, Dr. Daniel Rudman used recombinant GH in his study of people who were experiencing symptoms of aging. The group ranged in age from 61 to 81. In 6 months, the GH group showed an overall rejuvenation, including an 8.8 percent increase in lean body mass and a loss of 14.4 percent fat - without diets, exercise, or any change of lifestyle. The control group showed no change.

At approximately the same time, European researchers were studying people who had lost their pituitary glands due either to surgical removal or disease. Their findings were consistent with Dr. Rudman's: the control group that did not receive GH had a general slowing down of the system with overt signs of degeneration.

There are over 28,000 written studies reporting many positive results on human Growth Hormone. However, what plagued researchers most were the side effects of GH. It was Dr. Edmund Chein who solved the problem by devising a low dose (LD), high frequency (HF) system of GH therapy. Dr. Chein gave his patients a very low dose, once in the morning and once prior to sleep, six days a week. Given this way, the GH did not produce side effects.

14

sleep, six days a week. Given this way, the GH did not produce side effects.

From 1994 to 1996, Dr. Chein collaborated with Dr. Leon Cass Terry, a former associate of Dr. Daniel Rudman. They carried out a monumental study of 800 patients. With the low dose, high frequency approach, the results were amazing. To some degree, without knowing it, Dr. Chein and Dr. Terry's research was leading towards homeopathy.

HOMEOPATHY

HOMEOPATHY - HISTORY

Samuel Hahnemann, M.D., developed homeopathy in the early 1800s. The word "homeopathy" means, "like treats like." In other words, a symptom that results from taking a substance in its raw form can be alleviated by taking the same substance in a highly diluted and properly succussed, or shaken, form. This is somewhat like the vaccine principle.

According to the Arndt Schultz Law, substances vary in action depending on whether the concentration is high, medium, or low. High concentrations inhibit; medium concentrations suppress; and low, or minute, concentrations stimulate. When a substance is administered in homeopathic form, the concentrations work naturally and gently in the body.

HOMEOPATHY - NOW

Homeopathy has not only been recognized as a safe, effective way to help the body, but it is also the second most prominent form of medicine in the world. In fact, the Royal Family in England has had a homeopathic doctor for decades. Sales of homeopathics have risen 25 to 50 percent per year for several years, and even some insurance companies have begun to cover homeopathic treatments. Homeopathics have been used successfully to treat various physical and emotional problems and are also very effective when used topically.

Homeopathy encourages the body to clear itself. In contrast allopathic, or modern, medicine artificially and forcefully suppresses symptoms of disease and is sometimes toxic to the body. There is no toxicity associated with homeopathics since they use minute amounts of a substance and encourage the body to bring itself into balance. Compare this to the fact that over 100,000 people are known to have died in 1997 from using pharmacological drugs!

HOMEOPATHIC POTENCY AND PREPARATION

Homeopathic potency is important: it first tells us how a homeopathic product is made at the lab, and then tells us how it will work. There are two common types of potency: the decimal potency, denoted by an "X" (10), and the centesimal potency denoted by a "C" (100). A decimal potency is prepared as follows:

<u>Growth Hormone</u>   <u>Base</u>
1 part   **9** parts

A base is typically made of purified water, alcohol, glycerin, lactose, or sucrose. Two or more of these ingredients are combined with the Growth Hormone and succussed, or shaken, (preferably by hand) up to 100 times. This makes a 1X potency; we will call it the "New Potency."

Another 1 part of this "New Potency" is then combined with 9 parts of the base mixture and again succussed (preferably by hand) up to 100 times. This is a 2X potency. This process of dilution and succussion continues until the desired potency is reached. (A centesimal potency is prepared the same way, except that it is diluted 1 part to 99 parts.)

For a high quality product, it is important that the succussion be done by hand. As you can see, the process of hand succussing is not only time consuming, but also labor intensive. That is why some homeopathic manufacturers often use machines to succuss the product. This is a direct violation of homeopathy's strict guidelines. Dr. Hahnemann himself condemned the use of machinery in homeopathic preparation. Succussion by machine does not make a good quality product since the EMFs (electro-magnetic fields) or magnetic energies from the machinery can penetrate the remedies and distort their efficacy.

EFFECTIVENESS OF SMALL AMOUNTS

Years of research have shown that homeopathic remedies work similarly to their non-homeopathic counterpart but without the side effects. As a matter of fact, homeopathic remedies, down to simple minerals, are traditionally "proven" on test subjects. There are thousands of such tests in which healthy subjects are given doses of a particular substance, and all reactions are very carefully noted. The homeopathic "dynamized" version lines up with the non-homeopathic product.

The body itself breaks food down to microscopic amounts in order to transport nourishment to minute cells. For example, a thyroid hormone can be as small as 50 to 100 millionths of a gram in size. Despite the small size, bodily metabolism is maintained. Other hormones are even smaller, sometimes less than one trillionth of a gram.

Some scientists have finally discovered the homeopathic concept of minute dilutions. "Hormesis" is the term they use to describe *small doses* of substances that create a beneficial response. One cell biologist, Dr. Joan Smith Sonneborn states that "Hormesis appears to be a very real phenomenon" and further says it "may increase DNA repair...and...may also stimulate...the immune system, giving the organism greater protection against infection or chronic disease." Patricia Neafsey of the Tufts University School of Medicine and Harold Boxenbaum of the Merrell Dow Research Institute stated that "assessment of mortality data from modern day bioassay studies indicates the *low dose* (author's emphasis) animal exposure to a variety of toxic agents (homeopathy uses such "toxins" as arsenic and cadmium, etc. with great benefits) can, through an unknown mechanism induce beneficial changes which promote health and prolong life (longevity hormesis)." Put more simply, they are saying that a small amount works very well in promoting good health and a longer life!

18

HOMEOPATHIC GH

There is a growing belief that when Growth Hormone is combined with an oral homeopathic preparation, the results could be on the leading edge of anti-aging benefits. Remember: clinicians have found that smaller doses of GH work better and don't have side effects. Homoeopathists have known this for years! That is what makes the homeopathic GH concept so exciting. Only the positive therapeutic benefits manifest.

Many people already taking homeopathic GH have reported the same results as have those taking the molecular GH. But those results are obtained without the troublesome daily injections, at a substantially lower cost, and without the possible side effects a non-homeopathic dose could produce. This does not mean that homeopathic GH will substitute exactly for injectable GH, but it does offer an excellent, safe, convenient, more affordable and effective alternative.

Also, because of high dilutions, the homeopathic potencies of GH may make it even more effective in the body since scar tissue may not interfere with its absorption. In her best-selling book *Let's Get Well*, Adelle Davis, M.S., wrote that the presence of scar tissue in people's tissues and organs (including the liver and pituitary—the main source of GH) seemed to be the rule, rather than the exception. This could be another reason GH is not produced at acceptable levels in some persons. Even small scar tissue that forms in the pituitary can impede its production. Other factors which contribute to tissue and organ scarring include a lack of nutrients, diseases, nitrites, smoking (including second hand smoke), excessive alcohol intake, surgery, old internal wounds, high LDL cholesterol; the least known about is nerve impingement.

There is a growing belief that homeopathic doses of GH can penetrate better than non-homeopathic ones, particularly in the presence of scar tissue, and thus can possibly improve GH production in the pituitary and the immune system. Studies are now being conducted to prove this.

PROPER POTENCY OF GH

It is important to educate yourself. Read product literature and labels carefully, and understand what they mean. Some products state they are "homeopathic-like." Others claim they are "homeopathic" just because the formula contains minute amounts of an ingredient. Beware of both, since neither is a true homeopathic product.

Also, a product may have an "X" or a "C" after a number to show that a substance has been diluted, but it may not be a homeopathic, because it has not been properly succussed.

Some products give the number of "nanograms" (this is one billionth of a gram) of GH on the label and say, or imply they are "homeopathic." Again, this does not constitute a real homeopathic product. Homeopathic products are not measured in nanograms, grams or other similar measurements and you should not find this on the label of a truly homeopathic product - only the potency will be stated. Inquire as to how the product was prepared.

Research and homeopathic literature indicate that most of the favorable results with homeopathics have been with a fairly low potency, like 3X, 2C or 3C, or higher potencies, like 30X or 30C.

Homeopathic potencies for GH that range above 100 dilutions could have some benefit; however, many people really do not need such high potencies. There is also the strong chance that machinery was used to prepare these high potencies, because if these preparations were prepared by hand - as they should be - it would be very labor intensive to make them. Of course, some labs do produce higher potencies "by hand" only.

INTERESTING FACTS ABOUT HOMEOPATHICS

Consider that the following discoveries about homeopathics that may relate to the potentized GH. These facts show homeopathic substances are active - either in micro amounts or etheric (sub-atomic or deltron) levels.

- Trevor Cook, Ph.D. states that a magnetic resonance device detected subatomic activity in 23 homeopathic remedies.

- Dr. Emilio de Guidici says, "water molecules form structures capable of storing minute charges of electromagnetic signals."

- Dr. Wolfgang Ludwig, a German biophysicist, demonstrated that homeopathic substances give off measurable electromagnetic signals.

These researchers concluded that homeopathics demonstrate "energies" and that water molecules have a stable, hexagonal, lattice system, like an invisible honeycomb. This "honeycomb" can hold homeopathic "energies" and can change the structural shape of the water molecule lattice pattern! Succussing, or shaking, the homeopathic product seems to "transfer" the properties of the raw material to the water structure.

The British medical journal *Lancet* published an article on homeopathic remedies in 1997. The studies were double blind, which simply means that neither the researcher nor patient knew which product was the remedy and which was the placebo. There was also a randomized, placebo-controlled study in which the clinician randomly gave patients either the remedy or the placebo. The researchers concluded: "The results of our meta-analysis are not compatible with the hypothesis that the clinical effects of homeopathy are completely due to the placebo" (Linde, K. et al. "Are the Clinical Effects of Homeopathy Placebo Effects? A Meta

Analysis of Placebo Controlled Trials." Lancet 350:834-843, (1997)).

In other words, after all the trials were completed, the medical research showed homeopathy worked.

BENEFITS OF HOMEOPATHIC GH

- Homeopathics are gentle, safe and very effective.
- Growth Hormone is natural to the body; it is secreted by the pituitary gland. A person who uses homeopathic GH is not taking a material that is foreign to the body.
- Medical studies show that small amounts of GH taken at frequent intervals work better—which is also one of the basic principles of homeopathy.
- The homeopathic form of GH does not seem to interfere with any other remedy, supplement, or medicine that an individual might take.
- Homeopathic GH is more readily available and easier to use than injections.
- Homeopathic GH is much less expensive than injectable and oral molecular GH, both of which can cost hundreds of dollars per month.
- The homeopathic form of GH could gently encourage the pituitary to release and supplement GH—and balance the body. This is called homeostasis.
- Homeopathic GH products made of liquid are far superior to tablets, because liquid is easier to use and penetrates faster and more thoroughly over a larger surface area.

BENEFITS OF HOMEOPATHY

- According to homeopathic principles, the succussion process actually makes the GH potent, or dynamic, so it is even more bioactive in the body. The homeopathic process energizes *any* elements that are produced in this manner!

- The pituitary gland excretes GH at certain times, especially during the first 90 minutes of sleep. The body also times the release of GH. Molecular GH must be injected at certain times to try and mimic the GH pulsing. Since homeopathic GH is serially diluted, and potentized at successive levels, it continues to work in the body in a "time-release" manner. It doesn't matter when you take the homeopathic version. People could still get very good results if they wish to take GH at other than the suggested times.

- The homeopathic theory of dilution and succussion teaches that molecules can penetrate the cells more easily.

- Top quality homeopathic products are checked for purity both at the beginning and the end of the manufacturing process, thus assuring quality.

- Since the inception of homeopathy in the 1800s, no homeopathic remedy has ever been recalled because it harmed someone.

- Homeopathy is safe, effective and gentle, and an FDA ruling in 1938 is a testament to these features. The FDA has no "official" opinion on the efficacy of homeopathics, other than concern with safety, purity, ingredients and claims.

- Homeopathic factors seem to continue working in the body, even when someone does not take them every day.

- Over 200 years of research in homeopathy seems to show that it creates gentle, positive chain reactions, which promote general health.

Homeopathic Growth Hormone is not intended for those who have not yet completed their long-bone growth. Most people complete this phase between ages 20 to 25; however for some it occurs around age 30.

EXPECTATIONS FOR HOMEOPATHIC GH

Different people notice different results with homeopathic GH. Some people see immediate, dramatic results, while others experience more subtle benefits. With proper diet and exercise, the results can be faster, deeper, and more pronounced. Many people say they have begun a whole new life on GH therapy - you can, too!

Research shows that positive changes usually take place between one to six months, but can take up to one year. Have *patience!* Your GH levels may have been low for years. If your receptor sites are blocked, your body may need some time to respond in a positive manner.

If you smoke, drink, fail to exercise, or have a poor diet, the results you desire may take longer. You should also be aware that at certain times the body can shift into "neutral," and some results seem to diminish, or vanish altogether. If you experience this, your body may either be using GH to rebuild tissue or, to a degree, be resting. Experience indicates that, after a while, you should see a resumption of the benefits and even some vast improvements. This can be very exciting!

The following tables list some *general expectations*; they are based on worldwide clinical reports and research done with people who have taken injectable Growth Hormone. You may or may not experience these results with the homeopathic form (although experience seems consistent with this):

General expectations in the **first month** include:

Improved stamina	Vivid dreams
Better and sounder sleep, and feeling more refreshed upon awakening	More optimistic attitude and better sense of humor
Increase in energy	

General expectations in the **second month** include:

Improved muscle tone	Enhanced sexual function
Improvement in nail growth	Improvement to skin tone
Better digestion	Increase in strength
Weight loss	Better eyesight, including night vision

General expectations in the **third month** include:
Same as months 1 and 2 but probably heightened.
Some manifestations seem exceptional.

Mental processes improve, including desire to do and complete projects	Muscle size increases, especially if the individual works out
Faster recovery for wounds And muscle soreness	Hair growth
Reduction in PMS symptoms	Increase in sexual desire
Greater body flexibility	Less pain in joints
Alleviation of some menopausal symptoms	Improved nail growth (Sign of protein, nutrient assimilation)

General expectations in the **fourth month** include:

Same as above. Generally most improvements are heightened and are more consistent. Please note again that, at times, the body may shift into "neutral" and some results seem to diminish or vanish. Your body may be using GH to rebuild tissue or, to a degree, be resting. Experience indicates that, after a while, you should see a resumption of the benefits and even some vast improvements.

General expectations in the **fifth month** include:

Impressive weight loss and reduction of inches, since fat is reduced and muscle tissue is increased and toned	Improvement in skin texture and appearance (including lessening of skin discoloration)

Thickening of skin and greater elasticity	Reduction of the appearance of wrinkles
Thickening of hair, plus a shiny and healthy appearance	

General expectations in the **sixth month** include:
Same as above, but now better and with more consistent results. This could be the really exciting stage!

Cellulite greatly diminishes	Body is much more contoured
Eye sight greatly improved	Better emotional stability
Stronger resistance to colds, flu and other illnesses	Some pain and soreness disappear
Old wounds have healed or are healing	Excellent exercise tolerance
Grayed hair begins to return to natural color	
Medical tests show a reduction in cholesterol (LDL) and triglycerides, blood pressure normalizes, heart rate improves, some conditions that have been due to disease vanish or are diminished, and immune system improves.	

With proper diet and exercise, the results may be faster, deeper and more pronounced!

Keep in mind, if you take GH looking for dramatic results quickly, you won't be in line with the results of GH research which shows positive manifestation over 6 months to 1 year and longer. As previously stated, some people do notice immediate, dramatic results, while others experience more subtle benefits. Everyone is different; you must consider the condition you are now in and how long you have been in this condition. Whether you notice immediate results or not, according to experience, the GH is probably still working. Please continue to be faithful to your program. As GH injectable research indicates, results appear at three, six, and twelve months. One doctor says his patients "keep improving" year after year.

THE BEST WAY TO TAKE HOMEOPATHIC GH

Take GH drops under the tongue or use a spray under the tongue or on the walls of the mouth. According to homeopathic principles, it is recommended that food, toothpaste, chewing gum, coffee, mint, etc. be avoided for a half-hour before and after taking GH so there will be less likelihood of interference with the homeopathic action.

The best times to take GH are first thing in the morning, in the afternoon (around 4:00 to 6:00 p.m.) and last thing before going to sleep. Even if you take GH at other times, you should still receive great benefits. We suggest that you take GH five days a week, and skip two days, so the body's receptor sites can "rest." This will also enable the body to use the hormone and create its own. Occasionally (every 2 months), you may stop for seven days.

If you are sensitive to alcohol (which is often used in homeopathic products) or do not care for the taste, the drops can be placed in a small amount (3 ounces) of warm, not hot water for one minute to evaporate the alcohol. Remember that your body creates alcohol naturally. Dr. Hahnemann, the founder of homeopathy, suggested that another way for sensitive people to take homeopathic products is to apply the GH topically either to their wrists (undersides), stomach, face or chest.

Some researchers state that taking carbonated water with a supplement (such as amino acids) can enhance uptake of that supplement. Keeping this in mind, on occasion, you may want to take GH in one ounce of carbonated water, and see if you feel the difference. This should be done in moderation, as some health experts believe that carbonation should be taken only occasionally.

If the product is in a dropper bottle, avoid touching the dropper or liquid, if possible, limiting potential contamination. If your GH is in a spray bottle, it is best to avoid unscrewing the cap.

However, the alcohol or glycerin in many of the products acts as a good preservative.

Keep GH, and all supplements, away from extreme heat or light and away from drugs, toxic substances, x-ray, EMFs (electro-magnetic fields). This is just a precaution, since every substance has its limitations. Generally speaking, homeopathic ingredients are hardy and stable. Some homoeopathists report using homeopathics that were over 100 years old and still worked!

WHAT TO EXPECT

During the healing process, some people experience overt effects like a stronger heartbeat, headache, upset stomach, etc. You can easily reduce this by temporarily ceasing to take the GH or by reducing the amount of GH and taking it in water once a day or every other day in the morning or evening.

Sometimes, you may experience slight "aches and pains" in areas where you had old injuries. According to homeopathic principles, your body is "feeling" energy in an area where energy was previously blocked. This is called "retracing" or "aggravation." If symptoms are too strong, stop taking GH temporarily; or take less, and take it in water. When symptoms are relieved, and your body gets used to the "new" energy, you can slowly increase the GH to recommended amounts.

Take your time and "listen" to your body. The directions provided are *recommendations*. It is best to start *slowly*. Build up the amount of GH you consume and the *frequency* with which you take it, especially if you have any doubts about possible reactions to your present condition.

If you are a diabetic or have any medical condition, consult your doctor or holistic physician before taking GH or any supplement. Research shows that some diabetics on GH therapy decreased their need for insulin. This is good news, but a doctor should monitor your condition.

Be advised that any printed information is for educational and informational purposes only. Always consult an anti-aging health professional should the need arise.

WAYS TO ENHANCE GH AND
THE IMMUNE SYSTEM

The following are some things that can be done to possibly enhance GH in addition to taking homeopathic GH.

Amino Acids: It's true that these really are "the building blocks of life," especially for the immune system. They don't assimilate very well but amino acids are reported to be an excellent way to enhance GH in the body especially when taken in the homeopathic (liquid) or molecular (capsule) form. It's particularly good to take amino acid supplements first thing in the morning and just before falling asleep. An ounce of carbonated mineral water will help absorption. Different amino acids are known to work in different ways as follows:

- L-Arginine – boosts immunity and healing
- L-Glutamine – nourishes the immune system
- Aspartic Acid – enhances immune system and increases energy and stamina
- Alanine – aids overall immune function and blood sugar balance
- Full complex of 20-22 amino acids (in capsule form) assists general overall health.

Avoid Unhealthy Food, Drink and Habits: Poor nutritional habits contribute to aging and interfere with GH. Avoid drinking excessive amounts of alcohol and eating foods that are high in sugar and fat. Getting enough good quality sleep is also important to enhance GH.

Exercise: We all know the importance of exercise, but we don't always do it. Research shows that regular, systematic exercise done at least three times a week will boost the immune system, raise endorphin and enkephalin levels, improve the cardiovascular system, etc. Concentrated exercise raises GH levels because it stimulates the central nervous system; this empowers the hypothalamus, releasing a hormone that, in turn, causes GH release. Most people simply don't get enough exercise, which explains why so many are simply overweight and unhealthy.

Glandular Therapy: Either in the homeopathic or molecular form, glandular therapy can be an excellent way to consider boosting the immune system. Among several good glandular supplements for the immune system, three are especially good: liver, spleen and thymus. Remember that supplements are best in capsule form or in a liquid homeopathic form.

Supplements: A host of supplements are known to enhance the immune system. Some important nutrients are B-complex; vitamins A, C, E; and minerals like potassium, magnesium, selenium and zinc. Greens such as spirulina, chlorophyll, kelp and chlorella are also good. Both homeopathic and molecular ("food grown") supplements should be taken. C.A.W. or Catalyst Altered Water™ as formulated by Dr. John Willard (Willard Water) is an excellent therapeutic agent. Colostrum (capsules) is another wonderful immune system booster which contains natural IGF- I and other growth factors. Noni fruit (capsules) is currently an extremely popular product that is helpful for a wide range of conditions. Arctic root is new and a lot of studies confirm its powerful effect on the human system.

GH "ENHANCERS"

Non-homeopathic GH "enhancers" or "secretagogues," are nutrients designed to raise the production of GH in the pituitary; they do not contain GH themselves. While some people get good results with them, 30 percent of patients tested don't respond to these enhancers. GH enhancers have been around a long time and, in many cases, have never yielded the same quality and consistent results as actual GH.

There are now homeopathic enhancers, which seem to work well, however—especially when used with homeopathic HGH. They seem to work together in a multi-dimensional way. A homeopathic enhancer could also be effective when used alone because, due to the homeopathic action, the amino acids are readily assimilated.

You should be aware that (non-homeopathic) molecular enhancers could cost more because they require carrier ingredients to transport nutrients to the brain. Most enhancers contain amino acids, which can be poorly assimilated, making it difficult to penetrate the selective blood brain barrier.

Some people use molecular releasers, enhancers or secretagogues to promote GH effectiveness. But when you use a non-homeopathic molecular enhancer or a releaser, you interrupt the body's natural feedback mechanism and speed up the receptor sites that are ready to bind to the GH. The receptor sites remain in a state of high stimulation and do not have time to rest. For that reason, some authorities advocate "cycling" molecular GH releasers, or taking them for briefer periods, with set intervals of rest. The same applies to the injectable GH.

TECHNICAL INFORMATION

Advanced Information about the Pituitary and Its Related Functions

As you now know, Growth Hormone is secreted from the pituitary. The pituitary gland is about the size of a kidney bean and is divided by lobes, called the anterior and posterior. It is encased in a bony cavern at the base of the brain. The fact that the Creator saw fit to surround the pituitary in this protective cavern shows how valuable it is.

The anterior lobe creates and secretes several hormones, including vasopressin; but the most important one is Growth Hormone. Within the anterior lobe are specialized cells that produce GH - in fact; about half of this anterior lobe is comprised of such cells. The pituitary sends GH to the liver, and the liver then sends out IGF-I, or insulin-like growth factor-I, to do its work in the body.

The pituitary is under the direction of the hypothalamus, which is controlled by the central nervous system; the CNS, via another hormone, sends the GH into the body.

Scientists believe there is another hormone or neurotransmitter, yet to be identified, that stimulates the hypothalamus. The writer's speculation is the thalamus is probably involved somehow, and further research will reveal more about this "UFH," or "Unidentified Foremost Hormone."

DIAGRAM OF HGH FLOW

This diagram, which is greatly simplified, illustrates how GH is created and works in the system.

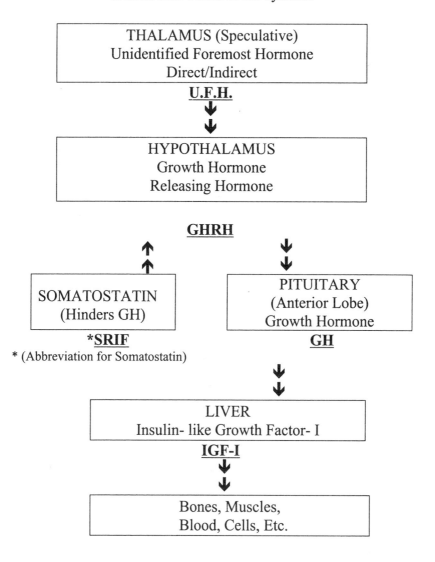

The author believes that the thalamus could be involved with an unidentified neurotransmitter or hormone that is created in the brain and, in turn, stimulates the hypothalamus to release

GHRH. The GHRH in turn motivates the anterior lobe of the pituitary to release Growth Hormone. Somatostatin is used by the hypothalamus to stop GH production when needed. GH then travels to the liver and causes growth factors- IGF-I and IGF-II (insulin-like growth factor I and II) to be released.

The wonderful benefits attributed to GH are the results of IGF-I and IGF-II activity.

IGF-1 (Insulin–like Growth Factor 1)

As you know, GH or Growth Hormone is excreted from the pituitary and from there it goes to the liver, which causes IGF-I or insulin-like growth factor I to be released. The liver also releases IGF-2, which works on renewal of the nervous system and other things.

IGF-I has similarities to insulin. It has balanced glucose metabolism and even helped clear insulin resistance in test subjects. IGF-I enhances protein metabolism and considering that our bodies constantly require protein, IGF-I is vital, especially if the pituitary has scar tissue, low-grade infection or is diseased (tumor, etc.) and cannot send GH out - at least in the needed amounts to maintain health.

The price for IGF-I is quite high at this time, but it is well worth the price. The homeopathic version of IGF-I proves to be the best in regards to cost and safety.

What does IGF-I do? Everything that GH does and more. As a matter of fact, there are even things that it does in the body that research has yet to reveal. The heart can be helped by IGF-I administration. In The New England Journal of Medicine, March 28, 1996 reports, "…growth hormone and IGF-I may contribute to improvements in cardiac performance…and can improve the efficiency of energy metabolism in the heart."

Studies with animals and different lab cultures show tremendous promise for everything from regenerating spinal cord motor neurons (150%-270%) to decreasing programmed cell death in chick embryos! In one case, IGF-I repaired and reconnected nerve endings that were up to 6 millimeters apart! Dr. Klatz states this is "a feat previously unheard of." People such as the actor Christopher Reeve could probably be helped by IGF-I's miraculous abilities to regenerate nerve damage. Dr. Klatz further says Swedish scientist Hans-Arne Hansson uses IGF-I and other growth factors to stimulate nerve regeneration. He also refers to researchers at Cephalon Inc. who say IGF-I may be the "long-sought endogenous motor neuron sprouting factor".

Phil Micans of International Aging Systems asserts that IGF-I is "ten times more potent than HGH"..." so possibly one would use less of it in dosing. IGF-I is a much smaller hormone being comprised of seventy amino acids as compared to HGH's 191.

Researchers have found that IGF-I can repair nerve damage. Nerve damage is very prevalent and can be caused from a number of things such as accidents, impinged nerves, poor nutrition, stress, disease, pollution, chemotherapy, etc. Since our nervous system powers all other systems in the body it is important we get the right nutrients like potassium, silica, zinc, and yes, IGF-I.

Phil Micans also predicts that IGF-I will be the "hormone of choice" in a few years. It's possible, he thinks, that a smaller dose of HGH will be needed to get the same anti-aging effects. There will always be a place for the other hormones and for GH, since it is the master hormone in control of the hormonal system.

Those few body builders that have obtained real recombinant IGF-I report muscle gains of 20 lbs. and more! The magazine, Muscle Media 2000, headlines IGF-I as "Possibly the Most Potent Body-Building Drug Ever!" The magazine article claims that some body builders report a 5% drop in body fat in one month! Increases in lean body mass and strength are described as "incredible". Some of these workout people are very excited about their results and are telling anyone who will listen.

Some body builders who court side effects by taking high doses of HGH, are also taking high doses of IGF-I, 50–100 micrograms per day as opposed to 10-50 micrograms, which is used normally. Taking homeopathic IGF-I could possibly eliminate this problem, as homeopathics have proven to be safe effective and reliable for the past 200 years.

Since HGH and IGF-I work so closely together in the body they could be an "unbeatable" team when used together as a homeopathic system. Growth Hormone seems to be a "night hormone" and IGF-I, a "day hormone" (one reason why both are needed), so the two could, as "supplements," work synergistically and catalytically in the body.

Although it is made with recombinant technology like HGH, it is presently hard to obtain. Unfortunately, most of the IGF-I that is purchased is fake. Again, it is important to know your sources.

There are products that claim they are "IGF-I" but are actually herbs and other ingredients. Read the labels carefully and do some studying. Most research and test results are based solely on just GH and IGF-I administration. The statement bears repeating, that a true GH product should have just GH or IGF-I as the **sole** active ingredient. However, both GH and IGF-I may be combined but, preferably in a homeopathic setting. Also, GH and IGF-I may be used in combination formulas as a "theme" such as Diet, Workout, etc.

IGF-II

Last, but certainly not least, is IGF-II. This important growth factor seems to work mainly on nerve cells. Nerve maintenance is vital and IGF-II is great at maintenance. Diabetic neuropathy affects about 15% of diabetics. The peripheral nerves break down over a period of time causing considerable pain; this can eventually lead to amputation and many health problems such as gastrointestinal disturbances. IGF-II could help in these tragic conditions. Scientists gave diabetic rats IGF-II and it prevented neuropathy. What is even more interesting is that even though their blood sugar was high the animal's health got much better!

IGF-I AND ALBUMIN

IGF-I uses albumin, a blood protein, which is created in the liver and is composed of 52% carbon, 23% oxygen, 16% nitrogen, 7% hydrogen, and 1.5% sulfur. Very few, if any, popular books on HGH discuss albumin and HGH, which play a vital role in the maintenance of body functions and health.

IGF-I utilizes albumin for many bodily functions, some of which are:

- Control of cellular moisture
- Cellular development and restoration
- The movement of nutrients to cells and waste extraction
- Assisting in the complete digestion of food
- Wide range of anti-oxidant activity
- Balancing blood pH and blood stabilization

Stress can minimize albumin levels and interfere with GH activity as well as your entire well-being, including vital energy production.

MEASURING GH USING IGF-1

We know GH triggers IGF-I release in the liver. Therefore, IGF-I is one way to measure GH production. Earlier thinking proposed that the ideal IGF-I level was 350 ng/ml in the blood. Some researchers have found that the 350 ng/ml doesn't apply to everyone. These researchers state that some people have IGF-I levels of 250 and less, yet are "normal" when tested for overall health performance, etc. This goes along with the homeopathic model, which stresses that individual balance is achieved with dynamized, tiny amounts of a substance like GH. Thus, using homeopathic GH may or may not raise IGF-I levels; in fact, the levels may even (temporarily) drop somewhat. Later that level will normalize or move to a level that is appropriate for each individual if they keep taking GH. This latest finding seems to confirm homeopathic research, which shows that symptomatology, may be cleared, yet the serum levels may not always coincide with "accepted" levels.

Adelle Davis, M.S., reported that some people require high amounts of certain nutrients; but when other nutrients are taken, those same "high" amounts" can be reduced because a booster or utilization effect takes place. For example, once mineral levels are "normal" for that person, many other vitamin dosages can be lowered. Muscle building is another example of the "down before up" homeopathic principle. When we work out, the muscle tissue is broken down to some extent. The "soreness" we feel later is the body repairing the tissue in order to build toned and larger muscles- "down before up".

The Importance of Vitamin E and GH

There is more vitamin E concentrated in the pituitary than anywhere else in the body. If the pituitary is to be healthy, it must have plenty of Vitamin E. Some health experts recommend taking a homeopathic form of vitamin E as well as natural ("food grown")

38

supplements to improve body function, decrease scar tissue, and increase GH processing.

Many people do not get adequate nutrition. To make matters worse, as we age, there is a significant loss of HCL and digestive enzymes. We also suffer damaging effects from pollution, chemicals, stress, and a decrease in exercise. The individual is less and less able to digest food as thoroughly as they should. This leads to sluggish GH secretion by the pituitary.

The problem is two-fold: the person's diet simply doesn't supply enough Vitamin E, and what they do get is not fully extracted. In her book, *Let's Get Well*, Adelle Davis, M.S., says that if a person does not get adequate amounts of Vitamin E, scar tissue can form over a period of time in different parts of the body. It can form in the liver, for instance, and interfere with bodily functions. In their book, *Life Extension*, Shaw and Pearson concur; they explain that GH stimulates IGF-I (also called Somatomedin C) in the liver. However, if a liver is scarred, it may not produce enough IGF-I to maintain youthful energy and health. In homeopathy, calcium fluoride 6X (or higher) is used to improve elasticity and reduce scar tissue as it converts to hydrofluoric acid.

The Importance of Chiropractic Adjustments and GH

Another critical factor is based on the innovative work of Dr. B.J. Palmer, the developer of chiropractic. During the 1920s and '60s, Dr. Palmer used various instruments, including an electronic device, to measure brain waves to the body. This device could detect nerve impingements, which reduced nerve energy to different parts of the body, including the hypothalamus. Remember: the hypothalamus controls the pituitary, which, in turn, releases GH and other chemicals.

Dr. Palmer knew that the hypothalamus was connected to the central nervous system and the nervous system itself rules all other systems in the body (Gray's Anatomy). Dr. Palmer believed one should look to the nervous system for the cause of disease; he called it "dis-ease" - not at ease! He discovered that pressure, especially in the neck vertebrae, could encroach on the nerves, (and we now know) affect GH release, and possibly even cause disease. By adjusting, especially, the Atlas vertebrae, through which some 427 trillion nerves pass in the neck, the pressure would be relieved; the body could function better and release GH properly. Dr. Palmer's Palmer Toggle Recoil Method (formally called HIO), a form of chiropractic adjustment, is a seemingly effective way to help the body release GH. Instrumentation and over 70 years of research back this method. The full spine may be corrected also.

GH COMMON QUESTIONS, MISCONCEPTIONS, AND CONCERNS

- **Is all GH alike?**

   No. Make sure the GH you take is somatotrophin or HGH which has the identical structure of human GH. The source of GH should not be porcine (pig), bovine (cow), or other animal products. Just because the label or brochure says GH, or Growth Hormone, doesn't mean it is recombinant human GH.

- **What if I stop taking GH? Will I instantly "age"?**

   No. As the effects of the injectable GH eventually wear off, "normal" aging will continue, but once a person has taken GH and seen the results, s/he generally wants to continue taking it. The same could be said of the homeopathic version.

   There are supplements everyone should take throughout life for health maintenance. Homeopathic GH is affordable, so you don't have to worry about not being able to continue taking it.

- **Is it possible to take too much *homeopathic* GH?**

40

It is possible to take too much of anything, including food and water! Homeopathic GH is gentle and safe. The amount that constitutes "too much" varies from person to person, depending upon the individual's condition. However, if a person took "too much" over a long period of time, they may or may not experience temporary negative or uncomfortable symptoms.

Reducing the amount of GH taken, or temporarily discontinuing the GH, easily alleviates these symptoms. When symptoms subside, the dosage can be gradually increased.

- **Will GH interfere with medications, herbs, etc.?**

The homeopathic form of GH does not seem to interfere with any medications or other substances, including supplements. In fact, your supplements may work more effectively when you are taking GH. If you are taking stimulatory drugs or herbs, such as ginseng, *gradually* increase your GH; you don't want to add "power to power."

- **Does GH have side effects?**

Most side effects that have been reported occurred with injectable GH. When we consider all the worldwide GH studies, we see that the few side effects that did occur resulted from too high a dose of injectable GH and from taking it either at the wrong time, or at incorrect intervals.

Dr. Chein and Dr. Terry have treated thousands of people with GH and found that they eliminated side effects by administering a low dose first thing in the morning and last thing in the evening. They followed this plan consistently, six days a week, and allowed one-day off so the receptor sites could relax and the body could create and process the GH. With this carefully prescribed method, there have been few, if any, side effects.

Also, homeopathic GH has been diluted at successive levels and hand-succussed, or potentized, at each of those levels. This greatly reduces the chance of side effects while possibly increasing the effectiveness of GH. The homeopathic process has proven itself worldwide for around 200 years.

Some people may experience slight "detoxification" effects or temporary "tiredness". Therapeutic homeopathic agents encourage the body toward health without artificially suppressing symptoms. If you experience uncomfortable detoxifying, stop or reduce the frequency and dosage until the effects pass (two to three days or longer), and drink lots of distilled water. You may put a reduced amount of GH in water, but be sure to replace the water-soluble vitamins, such as B complex and vitamin C, since copious amounts of water can flush them out of the body.

Sometimes, the body "retraces," or experiences a past health condition or an old injury. When this happens, the body is "cleansing" itself of that past condition. This is normal and should disappear in a few days or weeks, depending on your condition. This is similar to detoxification and should be handled as such.

- **Can GH cause cancer or speed up cancer?**
Dr Chein and Dr. Terry treated nearly 1,000 people who were at risk for cancer, and not one developed cancer! In fact, one man with prostate cancer actually had his cancer disappear with GH therapy. In the 28,000 studies on GH, the cancer risk factor does not seem strong when proper dosage, timing, and spacing of injections were administered.

Dr. Ronald Klatz is one of the world's top experts on GH and President of the American Academy of Anti-Aging. He carefully studied this area and concluded that GH gives a "protective effect," because it "revives and rejuvenates the immune system."

- **Does GH harm the organs of the body like the heart or liver?**
Some patients who received correct doses of injectable GH experienced a re-growth of their organs, and the organs functioned

better than they had for a long time. The same holds true with animal studies. Dr. Keith Kelly found that the thymus gland, a vital part of our immune system, shrinks as we age; with GH, the thymus actually goes back to its original size. Again, overdosing and giving GH at the wrong time can cause problems. But even these symptoms disappear when dosage and timing are adjusted, or if the procedure is terminated.

Some studies have shown that GH actually strengthens the heart. Others show that some damaged or diseased livers and other organs have been brought back to a state of health with GH therapy.

- **Does GH cause carpal tunnel syndrome and edema?**
    Injectable molecular GH, administered in doses that are too high, can cause these two prominent symptoms. However, it must be noted that when the GH dosage was reduced, or if the treatments were discontinued, the symptoms disappeared after about two to three weeks. If the GH dose is too high, then too much water can collect in parts of the body and cause edema or carpal tunnel syndrome. Once again, homeopathic GH should not produce these symptoms because of the minute, specially potentized amounts.

- **Does a doctor need to inject GH?**
    We recommend that a doctor administer the molecular (injectable) form of GH, although Dr. Chein and Dr. Terry, and other doctors have taught their patients to inject themselves twice a day. Technically, the molecular GH is the only kind of GH to be administered by a trained, medical professional. No doctor is needed to administer homeopathics. The FDA does not control homeopathics, except when false or misleading claims are made, or purity or ingredient violations arise.

- **Will Homeopathic GH cause tissue, bones and organs to grow abnormally large?**

No. Problems of this sort arise only if injectable molecular GH is used in too high a dosage over a prolonged period of time. Using injectable, full molecular (not homeopathic) GH in excess could cause some increase in tissue or bone size unless   the injection dosage is reduced or stopped.

Dr. Klatz deplores "deliberate and continuous overdosing" of injectable GH. *Anything used in excess can cause side effects*. As stated, Dr. Chein and Dr. Terry found that GH given in low doses is extremely safe. Homeopathic GH is a micro dose amount that is even lower than Dr. Chein's and Dr. Terry's dosage. This greatly reduces the chance of any kind of side effects.

- **What is oral molecular GH, a product taken sub-lingually, and does it need a special compound to get into the body?**
   Some formulas use several ingredients called "chaperones," carrier ingredients, or a "polymer matrix" to help the body absorb and enhance the GH. This increases the cost of the product and isn't necessary with homeopathic GH. It is intrinsic to the nature of homeopathics not to need a "penetration" compound.

Homeopathic research has proven repeatedly that, because homeopathics are serially diluted and bioactived or succussed, they penetrate quickly and fully into the system. They can even be taken in water or on the skin with the same effect.

VARIOUS THEORIES OF AGING

"Youth is like virgin parchment, capable of any inscription."
— Massinger
   Over the years, many researchers have developed their views of what causes aging. The Second Law of Thermodynamics states that everything is wearing down and our bodies follow this law as well. However, the idea is to slow the aging process down. After all, we will die, but let's not feel like we're doing it for years! The American Academy of Anti-Aging Medicine has listed

at least nineteen different theories why people age. They are condensed here for the sake of brevity.

The "Wear and Tear" Theory

August Weisman, a German biologist in 1882, stated that aging was caused by overuse and abuse of toxins in the environment, diet (high in fat, alcohol, nicotine, sugar, etc.), and emotional stresses. HGH will help the body function more efficiently, but "abuse" needs to be curtailed.

The Neuroendocrine Theory

Dr. Vladimir Dilman believed the neuroendocrine system, under the direction of the hypothalamus, begins to exert less of an influence on our system and the positive healthy action it helps create begins to lessen. Even the depletion of one hormone can start the downward spiral of aging. By replacing these hormones, especially HGH, we can, according to some researchers, reset the balance of hormones thus promoting body balance.

The Genetic Control Theory

This postulate focuses on the DNA in our cells and asserts that we are "programmed" to get old, sick, and then die. We now know we're not limited by genetics. We have some opportunity to give our cells the kind of nutrition and exercise that our bodies need, thus extending our lives and improving our health. GH factors in this equation can greatly improve the quality of life in spite of the DNA -"Death is Near Always" -philosophy.

The Free Radical Theory

In 1954 R. Gerschman introduced, and Dr. Denham Harman then developed, the "Free Radical Theory." This states that molecules that hold a free electron (a free radical) can and do react with other molecules and cause not only toxicity but also damage to bodily organs, including the skin and hair. Once again, we can reduce this "free-radical" damage by taking certain nutrients, including antioxidants like Vitamin C, E, etc. GH will also help to minimize free-radical damage by straightening out the body's system.

Waste Accumulation Theory

This theory has our cells producing waste products that, over time, cannot be successfully eliminated. So toxins build up, and finally interfere with normal cell metabolism, thus destroying cellular function. Nutrition, good diet, GH supplementation, proper rest, and exercise can greatly reduce this toxic state of affairs. As always, one must reduce stress and live as stress-free as possible. Also, there are some excellent detoxification programs that will fight this excess accumulation.

Limited Number of Cell Divisions Theory

Cell division turnover is deeply affected by the accumulations of cellular waste. An older person's cells divide fewer times than a young person's cells; because the latter divide more rapidly, they are able to handle the toxic waste in the body much better. Research shows GH will help normalize cellular division.

Hayflick Limit Theory

Drs. Hayflick and Moorehead in 1962 proposed that a sort of biological "clock" within each cell mediated aging. Cells have limitations on their life span. Some divide about fifty times in this life span, and then cease. Cells that are well nourished divide about fifty times a year. Cells that lack proper nourishment take up to three times as long to divide. The message: cells should be "fed" with the proper nutrients so they can divide properly and reach their full growth potential. Proper cellular function requires HGH at healthy levels since GH drops about 14% every ten years after we reach twenty-one to thirty-one years of age.

Death Hormone Theory

In the view of endocrinologist Donner Denckla, a "death hormone," DECO (a decreasing consumption hormone) released from the pituitary causes a loss of neurons. Dr. Denckla removed the pituitary glands in test rats and found that their immune and cardiovascular systems greatly improved. Denckla felt that aging causes the pituitary to release DECO, which causes a drop in the amount of thyroxin and slows down the metabolism, thus speeding up the aging process. This is why some researchers believe it's vital to supplement HGH for a healthy pituitary gland thus reducing the DECO factor.

Thymic – Stimulating Theory

Dr. Alan Goldstein asserts that the thymus gland is the "master" of the immune system. We do know that it shrinks with age from about the 200 gr. range to about 3 gr. by the age of 60. The theory assumes that when the thymic capacity, including its work with hormones, slows down, the body begins to weaken and aging quickens. Dr. Keith Kelly and others have shown that GH actually enlarges the thymus (and other glands) thus rejuvenating the immune system.

Mitochondria Theory

The mitochondria in cells help produce ATP, our main energy source. But free radicals are formed and mitochondria are susceptible to attack, thus leading to damaged DNA and causing disease and aging. Taking antioxidants and a GH program could aid in mitochondria repair.

Errors and Repair Theory

Dr. Leslie Orgel has stated that the body's process for creating protein in the cells is crucial, and disaster can strike if there are any "errors." Making proteins and DNA is not always done properly, so the body attempts to repair the errors. However, the body does not make those repairs as perfectly as it should, and thus diseases, aging, etc., are the results. GH increases protein synthesis and bodily repairs (as when we are young) but GH decreases with age. Supplementation of GH would certainly be in order according to over 28,000 research papers worldwide.

Redundant DNA Theory

Dr. Zhores Medvedev affirms that life span is contingent upon the degree of properly repeated gene sequences. Accumulated gene error is the culprit in this theory and states there are "genes in waiting" with the same erroneous DNA that are used until the system is broken down. Again, GH could hold some very positive answers in assisting proper gene sequences.

Cross-Linkage Theory

In 1942 Johan Bjorksten blamed cross-linking for premature aging and disease. Cross-links are needed in proteins for tone and strength, but the wrong kind of cross-links can cause wrinkled skin, artery hardening, etc. The exchange and transfer of nutrients is blocked or slowed down thus perpetuating cellular damage, disease, and aging. Free radicals and other substances contribute to cross-linkage. Exercise, good diet, and having a good supplementation program with GH has shown good results in slowing cross-linkages.

Autoimmune Theory

The immune system is our main defense against disease and aging. With age, the immune system sometimes cannot distinguish between antibodies and proteins and actually fights itself. One example is the dreaded lupus disease. According to GH research immune system function can, in some cases, be enhanced.

Calories Restriction Theory

Dr. Roy Walford believes that a high nutrient low calorie diet along with supplementation and exercise will retard the aging process. Weight would be lost slowly until that person's metabolism normalizes, thus creating an environment conducive to health and longevity. He has developed a special diet conforming to his theory. HGH improves digestion, nutrient utilization and burns fat and builds muscle.

Gene Mutation Theory

Since the 1940s, researchers have delved into mutations and the aging process. Genes experience mutations, which concern life itself. Radiation was used to prove mutations lessened health and life span. Later it was shown that radiation in tiny amounts increases animal life span. It seems homeopathic principles such as the "minute dose" keep getting confirmed - "a little goes a long way." Experienced researchers have found that, directly and indirectly, HGH is behind all the bodily processes including proper genetic function.

The Rate of Living Theory

In 1908 physiologist, Max Rubner, propounded the concept that each person has a certain amount of energy. If this energy ticks off slowly, then we age gracefully. If our energy is used up at too rapid a pace, then the aging process *transpires* too rapidly. GH research indicates that proper levels of Growth Hormone cause the body to create the right amount of energy.

Order to Disorder Theory

There is order in a healthy young person, but after sexual maturity, the energies that caused this order begin to diminish. The well ordered system of things begins to break down, causing *molecules* to create errors that are passed on to other molecules, etc. This process is what is behind the aging process. Some scientists reason that once Growth Hormone levels start to fall, a "breakdown" process begins and negative aging sets in.

The Telomerase Theory of Aging

Telomeres are nucleic acids (in sequence) attached to chromosomes. The telomeres help keep chromosomes "healthy." With cell division they are shortened causing damage and aging. There is an enzyme called a "telomerase" which can build up our telomeres. Rebuilding telomeres is a goal in some research circles (Adapted from Journal of Anti-Aging medicine ; Drs. Klatz and Goldman).

All of these theories have some problems; but perhaps they all, to some degree, explain aging. We can conclude that....

- Maintaining a vigorous nervous system is the key to slowing the aging process.
- One must eat nutrient rich, unrefined food with digestive enzymes/HCL (five small meals is best).
- One should get the right amount of sleep and exercise.
- A good supplementation program involving HGH stimulation is vital, since many researchers believe a diminished GH supply is associated with disease and aging.
- Last but not least, monitoring the highest quality of thoughts –"your body is your mind condensed." We all know what negative thoughts can do to our emotions; imagine how they impact our health. *"As a person thinks in their mind so shall they be"—Proverbs.*

CONCLUSION

Medical studies seem to show that the aging process is related to a decrease in Growth Hormone. By supplementing GH, we may be able to control, and possibly reverse, the aging process.

GH has been used for many years. In 1985, "recombinant" Growth Hormone was developed - and it revolutionized the GH world. Recombinant GH is made from non-human, 'natural' elements and is identical to human Growth Hormone. Early side effects with injectable GH were mainly due to dosages that were too high and being taken at the wrong time. Interestingly enough, the best results were obtained with the smallest dosages of GH. Without knowing it at the time, studies were pointing to the effectiveness of homeopathy!

Homeopathy may take GH to the safest, most sophisticated and effective level ever seen. Combined with years of scientific research along with the benefits, safety and effectiveness of 200 years of use of homeopathy.

For the *first* time, the author would like to advance the concept that homeopathic Growth Hormone could be a Universal Agent—i.e., one product that can help many different conditions in the body. One of the reasons for this assertion is that no matter what old condition someone has had, the homeopathic GH seems to "retrace" it from the most recent appearing condition back, in order, to the oldest conditions. This "retrace" or "aggravation" lasts a short while; it is basically gentle and does disappear, leaving the person with apparent relief. So far, this phenomenon is consistent no matter what condition one has had in the past.

By putting homeopathic manufacturing processing together with GH, it seems that almost anything may be possible.

Advanced research in both the medical and natural health fields point to GH as a valuable treatment. The old homeopathic process could bring HGH, IGF-I and IGF-II into new realms and very safe ones at that. How exciting to be on the leading edge of anti-aging and begin *Feeling Younger with Homeopathic HGH!*

FOUR TESTS – "BIO MARKERS" OF AGING

There are four tests, as mentioned by Roy Walford M.D. in his book, *The 120 Year Diet: How to Double Your Vital Years* (as mentioned in *Grow Young with HGH*, by Dr. Ronald Klatz).

1. Skin Flexibility Test:

As you age, you lose elastin and collagen along with skin moisture, and the skin becomes less elastic. GH tones the skin, and a lack of GH could be one indicator of sagging, inflexible skin. To test your skin's resiliency, use your thumb and forefinger to pinch the skin on the back of your hand for 5 seconds

You must time how long it takes the skin to go back to its normal place. Here are rate times (note: time will vary):

   a. Forty-five and fifty Years- 5 seconds
   b. Sixty Years- 10-15 seconds
   c. Seventy Years- 35-50 seconds

2. Stationary Balance Test

This is an important test which checks how much time you can stand on one leg with closed eyes before you fall. Stand with both feet together on a flat non-carpeted area. You can wear flat shoes or be barefooted. Have someone there to keep you from falling.

Now with eyes closed lift your foot (left foot if you are right handed—right foot if you are left handed) about 6 inches above the floor with your knee bent at a 45-degree angle. Stand still.

The person helping you needs to time how long you can stay in this "holding pattern" without opening your eyes or falling. This test should be done three times to get an average time. A person in their 20's will be able to do this for about 30 seconds on average whereas an older person usually falls in about 4-8 seconds.

3. Vision Reaction Test

Get a magazine or newspaper and hold it with your arms extended. Very slowly (without any glasses) bring the magazine or newspaper towards your eyes until the normal-size print begins to blur.

Have your partner measure the distance between your eyes and the printed matter. Here is the average:

  a. Twenty year-old - about 4 inches
  b. Thirty year-old - about 5.5 inches
  c. Forty year-old - 9 inches
  d. Fifty year-old - 15 inches
  e. Sixty year-old - 39 inches

4. Ruler Test

This is to test reaction time. Take an eighteen-inch ruler (wooden) and get a partner to hold the ruler at the top with the eighteen-inch mark at the bottom with your fingers in between. Use your dominant thumb and middle finger which should be three and a half inches apart (equally on both sides of the ruler) at the eighteen inch point. Your partner is to drop the ruler without telling you and you try to catch the falling ruler. Do this procedure three times and get an average.

Illustration: Here are the averages for people in their twenties and sixties:

  a. Twenty year-old - 11 inch marker
  b. Sixty year old- 6 inch marker

MEASURE YOUR GH PROGRESS

You may use this form to chart your progress while using homeopathic GH. For the first month, your body may be in a state of acclimation to the GH properties, therefore, you may want to copy this form to continue tracking the following months. We suggest this value system to chart your weekly program.

1 = poor   2 = poor/fair   3 = fair
4 = good/excellent   5 = excellent

Present Condition	MONTH 1			
	WEEK1	WEEK2	WEEK3	WEEK4
Energy Level				
Sleep				
Mental Attitude				
Memory				
Mobility				
Weight				
Hair				
Skin				
Eyesight				
Health Conditions				
Past Health Conditions				
Present Injuries				
Past Injuries				
Nails				
Muscle Tone				
Sex				
Digestion/ Elimination				
Healing/Recovery				
Urinary System				
Allergic Reaction				
Cold/Flu Frequency				

TESTIMONIALS

The following is a small sampling of the positive benefits many people have experienced with homeopathic GH. Of course, everyone is different, and no promises or claims are made. But certainly, good things are being reported, and many individuals are quite pleased with their results.

"My wife and I have been using.... [Oral homeopathic HGH].... for sometime now, and I have been supplying them to my 94 year old aunt. We are receiving all the benefits we were previously experiencing with the injectable form of HGH and at a greatly reduced price. As you know, I have been taking the HGH injections....longer than any other adult we know of. I have been called the "Father of Growth Hormone" by the media, based on my having pioneered the field, and have appeared all over the world promoting the use of HGH as a necessary anti-aging medication...."

—Howard Turney, Founder of the first
Growth Hormone clinic for purposes of
rejuvenation

"Health and beauty are important to me. Homeopathic Growth Hormone has helped me keep my weight down, improve muscle tone, stabilize my energy, and improve my skin quality. With my busy schedule of traveling, speaking and taking care of my family, it is important that I look and feel healthy."

—Sheri Rose Shepherd,
Mrs. United States, 1994

"After I began taking homeopathic Growth Hormone I noticed more energy, better sleep and I lost about 18 pounds. As time went on my fingernails began to grow faster, and my eyesight (nearsighted) improved drastically. My hair is growing back and is changing to its natural color. All this in only 6 months - I can't wait to see what else happens in the future."

—William Mason, Ph.D.

"When I began taking homeopathic HGH, I felt my energy level increase within a few days. After several weeks I was aware of enhanced muscle mass, which helped me to increase my exercise and activity level as I had hoped. As a 50-year-old man, I sincerely appreciate a product that supports my wellness and, of course, helps me to feel and look younger."

—A. Renaud, Marketing Executive

"I see sharper...I hear better... with a sense of improved smell too... I sleep much better...my energy is definitely elevated; I have lost six pounds, gained harder muscles...my hair seems darker, thicker and stronger, plus there is major improvement in the texture, tone, and elasticity of my skin. Facial wrinkles have disappeared."

—Y. Bendarzewski, Architect

BIBLIOGRAPHY

Boericke, Wm. M.D., *Homeopathic Materia Medica*. Philadelphia, PA, Boericke & Runyon, (1927).

Boxenbaun, H. Neafsey, PJ, Fournicer,DJ. Hormesis, Gompertz. Functions, and Risk Assessment. Drug Metabolism Review 19: 195-229, 1998.

Brewitt, Barbara, Ph.D. "HIV-AIDS Clinical Homeopathic Trial Status / Summary of Clinical Studies on HIV". Biomedical Exploration, LLC / Biomed Comm Inc. (June 1997).

Davis, Adelle, M.S. *Let's Get Well*. New York: The New American Library, Inc., (1972).

Demarco, Carolyn, M.D. "Anti-Aging Breakthrough—Homeopathic Growth Factors." Let's Live, (March, 1998).

Gelato, M.C. MD, Ph.D. Aging and immune function: A possible role for growth hormone. Hormone Research, (1996) 45:46-49.

Hickey, R.J. Radiation Epidemiology, Extrapolation, and Opinion (letter). Chemical Engineering News, 23, pages 2 - 3. January 1989.

Iovino M. et al: Repetitive growth hormone-releasing hormone administration restores the attenuated growth (GH) response to GH—Releasing hormone testing in normal aging. Journal Clinical Endocrine Metabolism, 69:910 (1989).

Jamieson, J.; Dorman L.E. D.O. *Growth Hormone: Reversing Human Aging Naturally, The Methuselah Factor*. E. Canaan, CT: Safe Goods and Longevity News Network, (1997).

Kahn, C. "No More Slow Death." Longevity, February 1990.

Kelijman M: Age-related alterations of the growth hormone / insulin-like growth factor 1 axis. Geriatric Journal of American Society 39:295, (1991).

Klatz, R. D.O., M.D., *Grow Young with HGH*. New York: Harper Perennial, (1997).

Klatz, R. D.O., M.D., *Hormones of Youth*. Chicago, IL. Sports Tech Labs (1998).

Kunz, R.M., Jeffery, M.D. Editor. *The American Medical Association Family Medical Guide*. New York: Random House, (1982).

Marion, B., Joseph. *Anti-Aging Manual*. South Woodstock, Conn., Informative Pioneers, (1995; 1996).

Murray, Michael T. N.D. *Encyclopedia of Nutritional Supplements*. Rocklin, CA: Prima Publishing, (1996).

Palmer, B.J., Ph.C., D.C. *History in the Making*. Davenport, Iowa. Palmer College Press, (1957).

Pearson, Durk M.S. and Shaw, Sandy M.S. *Life Extension: A Practical Scientific Approach*. New York: Warner Books, (1983).

Phillips, L.S.; Harp. J.B; Goldstein, S; Klein, J; and Pao, C.I. Regulation and action of insulin-like growth factors at the cellular level. Proceedings of the Nutrition Society 49:451-458, (1990).

Prinz, Petal. Plasma growth hormone during sleep in young and aged men." Journal of Gerontology, 38:519, (1983).

Riley, D., M.D. "Proving/Homeopathic Study of Insulin–like Growth Factor I (IGF-1)", Integrative Medicine Institute, Santa Fe, New Mexico, (1997).

Rudman, D., M.D., et al. Effects of human growth hormone in men over 60 years old. New England Journal of Medicine, 323 (1990): 1-6.

Rudman, D., M.D. Growth hormone, body composition, and aging. Journal of the American Geriatrics Society 33 (1985): 800-07.

Rudman, D.; Kutnen, MH; Rogers, CM. Impaired growth hormone secretion in the adult population: Relation to age and adiposity. Journal of Clinical Investigation (1981): 67: 1361-1366.

Schwartz, Edward, Ph.D. "The Million Dollar Question— The Real Question in Homeopathy Is: Does a Substance That Has Been Repeatedly Diluted Really Work?" Health Way (March 1996).

Weiss, R. "A Shot at Youth". American Health, (Nov-Dec. 1993).

ANTI-AGING NATURAL PRODUCTS

HOMEOPATHIC GROWTH HORMONE: Dreamous Corp USA, 12016 Wilshire Blvd, #8, Los Angeles, CA 90025. 800 251-7543 or www.dreamous.com

BIO VITALE: Special conjugated water, homeopathic Noni, unique herbs and other products, 10 Corporate Park #130, Irvine, CA 92506. 949 851-9410, fax 949 851-9525

NATURAL HAIR COLORS AND COSMECEUTICALS: Herbaceuticals, Inc., 902-M Enterprise Way, Napa, CA 94558. 800 462-0666 or 707 259-6262.

FOOD GROWN VITAMINS AND SUPPLEMENTS: BioSan Laboratories Inc., P.O. Box 325 Derry, NH 03038. 800 848-2542

BIOAVAILABLE PLANT ENZYMES: Prozyme™ Products, LTD., 6600 N. Lincoln Ave., Suite 312, Lincolnwood, IL 60645. 800 522-5537.

CHLOROPHYLL PRODUCTS: DeSouza International, Inc., PO Box 395, Beaumont, CA 92223. 800 373-5171.

GREEN NUTRIENTS: Pines International, PO Box 1107, Lawrence, KS 66044. 800 697-4637.

INFORMATION RESOURCE: The American Holistic Health Association (AHHA), is a not-for-profit information clearinghouse. Information and resources concerning health publishers, companies, practitioners, and other health and wellness related groups that support a holistic style are available, free. AHHA, PO Box 17400, Anaheim, CA 92817-7400. 714 779-6152.

OTHER SUGGESTED BOOKS ON ANTI-AGING

Books By Sheri Shepherd,
Mrs. United States 1994
888 777-2439
Eating For Excellence;
Fit For Excellence;
Life is Not a Dress Rehearsal

Grow Young with HGH
By Dr. Ronald Klatz

OTHER BOOKS FROM SAFE GOODS

- Natures Secret Nectar NONI $ 4.95
- A.D.D. The Natural Approach $ 4.95
- The Brain Train $ 4.95
- El Metodo Natural (A.D.D. The Natural Approach Spanish)
                                                                $ 6.95
- The Secrets of Staying Young $ 9.95
- All Natural Anti-Aging Skin Care $ 4.95
- The Humorous Herbalist $14.95
- Plant Power $19.95
- Effective Natural Stress & Weight Management $ 8.95
- Natural Solutions for Sexual Enhancement $ 9.95
- The High Performance Diet $ 7.95
- A Guide To A Naturally Healthy Bird $ 8.95
- Plain English Guide to your PC $ 8.95
- The Backseat Flyer $ 9.95
- Nutritional Leverage for Great Golf $ 9.95
- The New Thin You $ 9.95
- Chronic Fatigue Syndrome for the Modern Woman $ 9.95
- Pycnogenol, The Bark with the Bite $ 8.95

AUDIO TAPES:

- A.D.D., The Natural Approach $ 9.95
- Crystalloid Electrolytes, Your Body's Energy Source $ 9.95

ORDER LINE (888)-NATURE-1, credit cards accepted
888 688-8731
Shipping: $4.00 each book/ Safe Goods, PO Box 36, E. Canaan,
CT 06024
Website: Safegoodspub.com